Balancing Hormones Naturally: A Woman's Guide to Herbal Remedies for Hormonal Health

Balancing Hormones Naturally: A Woman's Guide to Herbal Remedies for Hormonal Health

Copyright © 2024 by **Omolola Habib**

Table of Content

Introduction

Hormones play a profoundly important role in the overall health and wellbeing of women. These powerful chemical messengers regulate everything from metabolism and growth to reproductive function and mood. When hormones fall out of balance, it can have wide-ranging consequences for physical and mental health. All too often, women experience the exhaustion of adrenal fatigue, persistent anxiety and worry, sleep disruption, weight gain, low libido, menstrual difficulties, and more. These issues frequently have a hormonal component that goes overlooked.

Pharmaceutical hormone medications are commonly prescribed to try to rectify hormone imbalances. However, these synthetic hormones come with considerable risks and side effects. A more holistic, natural approach can often realign hormones gently and effectively. There are myriad natural ways women can support healthy hormone balance without negatively impacting overall wellness.

This book will explore the immense healing potential of herbs, foods, lifestyle changes and supplements for optimizing women's hormonal health. You will learn about the functions of key hormones like estrogen, progesterone, cortisol and thyroid hormone. Discover dozens of science-backed natural remedies that can safely moderate hormone levels, reduce troublesome symptoms, and restore your sense of wellbeing. From hormone-regulating herbs like maca and vitex, to anti-inflammatory foods and stress-busting self-care habits, this guide equips you with practical tools to bring your body back into balance.

Inside these pages, you will find:

- An overview of the female endocrine system and how hormonal communication regulates bodily processes

- The most common symptoms of hormone imbalance and its impact on mental and physical health

- Lifestyle tips for improving hormonal health through nutrition, exercise, stress management and more

- An extensive guide to healing herbs that gently modulate hormone levels and promote women's wellness

- Hormone-supportive foods, vitamins and supplements to incorporate into your diet

- Soothing practices to ease challenging hormonal transitions like perimenopause

- Natural solutions to address conditions like PCOS, endometriosis and menstrual problems

You were not meant to struggle with the effects of hormonal chaos. Whether you want to get to the root cause of troublesome symptoms, or proactively nourish balanced hormones for optimal health, this book will be your guide. Let's explore the many paths to hormonal wellbeing the natural way!

Chapter 1: Understanding Your Hormones

Hormones are like chemical messengers that travel throughout the body coordinating complex processes that keep us healthy. They are produced by the endocrine system, which includes glands like the pituitary, thyroid, adrenal, ovaries and pancreas. Hormones influence important functions like growth and development, metabolism, reproduction, mood and more.

Maintaining hormonal balance is crucial for overall wellbeing. When certain hormones become too high or low, it can lead to troubling symptoms. Hormone issues are extremely common in women due to fluctuations during menstrual cycles, pregnancy, perimenopause and menopause. This chapter will overview key female hormones, their roles in the body, and signs that they may be out of balance.

Key Female Hormones and Their Functions

Estrogen

Estrogen is considered the predominant "female" hormone, though it exists in both men and women. The three main forms are estradiol, estrone and estriol. Estrogen is produced mainly by the ovaries and is responsible for the development of female sex characteristics. It plays a vital role in reproductive health by thickening the uterine lining during the menstrual cycle to prepare for potential pregnancy.

Estrogen also impacts the brain, bone health, cholesterol levels, skin health and more. It can influence mood, regulating neurotransmitters like serotonin. Declining estrogen levels during perimenopause and menopause lead to symptoms like hot flashes, night sweats, vaginal dryness, irregular periods, mood swings and trouble sleeping.

Progesterone

Progesterone works together with estrogen in a delicate balance. It is secreted by the ovaries and by the placenta during pregnancy. Progesterone helps stabilize the uterine lining after ovulation each month. It is important for regulating menstrual cycles and preparing the body for childbearing.

During perimenopause, progesterone levels fluctuate irregularly leading to changes in menstrual flow. Low progesterone is associated with conditions like endometriosis and polycystic ovarian syndrome (PCOS). Balancing progesterone is also important for bone health and preventing osteoporosis in older age.

Testosterone

Testosterone is often considered a male hormone, but women's bodies also produce small amounts that affect metabolic processes, muscle and bone strength, sexual desire and pleasure. Testosterone begins declining in women from the 30s onwards. Excess levels of testosterone due to conditions like PCOS can cause acne, facial hair growth, male-pattern baldness and infertility.

Thyroid Hormones

Thyroid hormones T3 and T4 are produced by the thyroid gland and regulate metabolism, heart rate, body temperature, mood and digestion. Low levels cause hypothyroidism leading to unexplained weight gain, fatigue, hair loss, dry skin and feeling cold. High thyroid hormone levels result in hyperthyroidism with symptoms like rapid heartbeat, anxiety and unintentional weight loss.

Cortisol

Known as the main "stress hormone", cortisol is released by the adrenal glands. It helps regulate blood pressure, blood sugar and metabolism. Healthy cortisol levels follow a daily circadian rhythm and spike in response to stress. Excess cortisol from chronic stress disrupts sleep, immunity, mood, blood sugar regulation and more. This can lead to adrenal burnout.

Human Growth Hormone (HGH)

HGH is produced by the pituitary gland and as the name suggests, governs growth and cell regeneration. It promotes muscle and bone mass, and healthy body composition. Declining HGH levels with age lead to increased abdominal fat, less muscle tone, and weaker bones and joints. Low HGH also impairs collagen production resulting in sagging skin and wrinkles.

How Hormones Influence Health

When hormones are balanced and fluctuating appropriately, the body and mind function smoothly and effectively. Menstrual cycles progress normally, the mind is calm and focused, sleep is sound, and weight is well-managed. On the other hand, hormonal imbalances negatively impact both physical and mental health in numerous ways:

Physical effects:

- Irregular menstrual cycles and fertility issues

- Changes in sleep patterns and quality

- Unexplained weight gain or weight loss

- Loss of muscle mass and bone strength

- Hot flashes, night sweats

- Low libido

- Hair thinning/loss, skin changes

Mental and emotional effects:

- Mood swings, irritability, anxiety

- Depression

- Reduced motivation and focus

- Memory lapses and brain fog

- Low self-esteem

Hormone issues tend to worsen with age, especially for women approaching perimenopause and menopause. Fluctuating estrogen, declining progesterone, thyroid problems and high cortisol from stress create the perfect "hormone storm" - disrupting emotional stability, sleep, weight, energy levels and overall quality of life.

The good news is there are many safe, natural ways to gently restore hormonal balance without the use of synthetic hormones and medications. But first we need to understand the most common signs and symptoms associated with hormone imbalances.

Common Signs of Hormonal Imbalance

Here are some of the most common and bothersome symptoms that can signal your hormones have gone awry:

- Irregular periods and spotting
- Premenstrual syndrome (PMS) - bloating, cramps, acne, irritability
- Heavy or painful periods, clotting
- Anovulatory cycles - lack of ovulation
- Hormonal headaches and migraines
- Fatigue, low energy
- Hot flashes, night sweats
- Vaginal dryness
- Low libido
- Disrupted sleep
- Joint pain, muscle loss
- Weight gain or inability to lose weight
- Hair loss, thinning, dry skin
- New cognitive impairments like brain fog
- Anxiety, moodiness, depression
- Sugar and carb cravings

The more of these symptoms you identify with, the more likely hormone issues are at play. Identifying the root cause is the first step to addressing imbalanced hormones effectively. Common causes include chronic stress, thyroid disorders, low testosterone, perimenopause or menopause.

Now that you have a foundational understanding of key female hormones, their functions and how they profoundly impact wellbeing when imbalanced, we can explore the many natural ways to restore hormone health. The following chapters will provide lifestyle tips, describe healing herbs and foods, beneficial supplements and holistic solutions to bring your body back into balance. Get ready to feel renewed energy, calm and optimism as your hormone levels optimize in harmony!

Chapter 2: Lifestyle Tips for Balanced Hormones

The way we live each day has a tremendous impact on hormonal health. Making certain lifestyle adjustments can gently optimize hormone levels, often reducing or eliminating the need for medications. This chapter will explore science-backed habits for balancing hormones naturally.

Manage Stress with Self-Care

Chronic stress is one of the biggest culprits behind hormone chaos. The body is not designed to handle constant high cortisol levels. This causes dysregulation of reproductive hormones, thyroid function, blood sugar levels and more. Integrating self-care practices that activate the "relaxation response" are essential.

Try meditation: Just 10-15 minutes per day of meditation can lower cortisol and help restore hormonal balance. Meditation quiets mental chatter, lowers blood pressure, reduces inflammation and counteracts the effects of stress on the body.

Cultivate mindfulness: Being fully present throughout your day helps maintain lower stress levels. Practice mindful breathing, savoring your food, noticing nature and being fully focused on each activity.

Get a massage: Regular massages promote relaxation by increasing oxytocin and serotonin while decreasing cortisol and adrenaline. Massage also improves immune function and lowers inflammation.

Engage in hobbies: Do more of what you love! Gardening, painting, knitting and other hobbies you enjoy lower stress by focusing your mind on positive creative acts.

Go outside: Spend time in nature as often as possible. Forest bathing reduces cortisol, improves immunity and increases energy by exposing you to phytoncides from trees.

Listen to music: Soothing music promotes the relaxation response by slowing breathing and heart rate. Listen to classical, ambient or nature sounds to de-stress.

Laugh it off: Laughter really is great medicine when it comes to balancing hormones. Laughing for 10-15 minutes per day can significantly lower cortisol and adrenaline.

Get social support: Loneliness and isolation activate stress pathways. Spend time nurturing close friendships or join a social group to foster a sense of belonging.

Seek counseling: If emotional issues are exacerbating your hormonal imbalance, speaking to a therapist or counselor can help you process and release chronic stressors.

Consider adaptogens: These herbs like ashwagandha, rhodiola and ginseng help regulate cortisol, reduce anxiety and increase resilience to stress.

The key is to find activities that evoke your own relaxation response and make them a regular habit. This will go a long way in optimizing hormonal health.

Get Quality Sleep

Sleep has a major influence on hormone function. Lack of sufficient high-quality sleep dysregulates hormones and neurochemistry. Prolonged sleep deprivation leads to hormonal chaos:

- Increased cortisol and adrenaline
- Suppressed thyroid function
- Imbalanced reproductive hormones
- Elevated ghrelin increasing hunger and cravings
- Reduced leptin leading to carb cravings
- Increased risk of insulin resistance and weight gain

Aim for 7-9 hours nightly: Most adults need a minimum of seven hours, while eight or nine is optimal for robust hormone health.

Establish a sleep ritual: Unwind before bedtime through a calming ritual like Journaling, reading to enhance sleep quality.

Optimize sleep hygiene: Sleep in total darkness, keep your bedroom cool, avoid electronics before bed and use earplugs or an eye mask if needed.

Avoid caffeine: Eliminate caffeinated drinks after 2 pm so they don't interfere with your sleep.

Diffuse calming essential oils: Lavender, chamomile or clary sage essential oils promote relaxation and uninterrupted sleep when diffused before bedtime.

Take magnesium and zinc: These essential minerals reduce cortisol and encourage restful sleep. Take 200-400 mg magnesium and 10-15 mg zinc before bed.

Try sleep-supportive herbs: Herbs like passionflower, valerian, chamomile and lemon balm encourage better sleep quality when taken as a nightly tea or supplement.

Reduce alcohol: While alcohol may make you sleepy initially, it actually fragments sleep and alters REM sleep leading to less restorative slumber.

Quality sleep is just as important as diet and exercise for hormonal health. Make it a priority to get sufficient slumber to allow hormones to reset each night.

Incorporate Regular Exercise

Along with a healthy diet, regular exercise is crucial for keeping hormones balanced. All types of movement positively influence hormone function:

Aerobic exercise stabilizes blood sugar: This maintains proper insulin levels, reduces inflammation, helps regulate appetite hormones and encourages fat burning - especially beneficial for estrogen dominant issues like PCOS.

Strength training builds muscle, strength and bone density: This boosts testosterone levels, increases growth hormone production and prevents osteoporosis.

Yoga tones the endocrine system: Yoga poses stimulate hormone-producing endocrine glands and improve hormone receptor sensitivity.

Outdoor activity boosts vitamin D: Just 15 minutes of midday sun exposure increases vitamin D levels which are essential for hormonal health.

Aim for a combination of aerobic activity, strength training and gentle stretching like yoga or pilates for 30-60 minutes per day. Taking your exercise routine outdoors has added benefits. Spending time in nature, away from wifi and electromagnetic frequencies, also reduces cortisol.

Tips to make exercise a habit:

- Choose activities you enjoy - walking, dancing, hiking, cycling, etc.

- Exercise first thing in the morning to energize your day

- Workout with friends for motivation and accountability

- Try burst training: short bouts of intense exertion followed by recovery

- Add exercise equipment to your home - kettlebells, resistance bands, etc.

- Sign up for virtual classes when you can't get to the gym

Regular movement optimizes insulin sensitivity, helps maintain a healthy weight, reduces inflammation and keeps hormones balanced. Make exercise a priority for your hormonal health.

Avoid Hormone-Disrupting Chemicals

Everyday chemical exposures can wreak havoc on delicate hormone balance. These hormone disruptors mimic real hormones like estrogen, blocking receptors and altering the endocrine system. Avoiding these chemicals is key:

Avoid BPA: Found in some plastics, canned goods, and cash register receipts, BPA mimics estrogen and alters thyroid and testosterone function.

Avoid phthalates: These chemicals found in cosmetics, perfumes, plastics and food packaging reduce testosterone and thyroid hormones.

Reduce pesticide/herbicide intake: These mimic estrogen and have been linked to hormonal cancers and reproductive issues in women. Eat organic food as much as possible.

Avoid conventional personal care products: Opt for natural skincare, hair care, cosmetics, feminine care and body care products made without toxic ingredients.

Use natural household cleaners: Conventional cleaners contain chemicals that are hormone disruptors. Replace with green cleaners or DIY options like vinegar, baking soda and essential oils.

Filter your water: Tap water often contains toxins like atrazine, perchlorate and arsenic that disrupt endocrine function. Install a high quality water filter.

Ventilate your home: Off-gassing chemicals from furniture, carpets, paint and building materials act as hormone disruptors. Open windows regularly to ventilate.

The fewer hormone-disrupting chemicals you ingest or absorb through skin, the less taxed your endocrine system will be. Limiting chemical exposures supports overall hormonal harmony.

Social Connection & Nature for Hormone Health

Our hormones evolved to function optimally when we feel connected with others and are immersed in the natural world. Make these a priority:

Cultivate close relationships: Oxytocin, the "love hormone" is released when sharing affection, intimacy and closeness with others. Quality social ties reduce cortisol.

Bond with pets: Cuddling a dog or cat lowers cortisol and blood pressure. Pets provide unconditional affection and stress relief.

Join a group: Whether it's a book club or volunteer group, feeling a sense of belonging balances hormones.

Spend time outdoors: The sights, smells and sounds of nature balance cortisol, blood pressure and heart rate variability. Aim for 30-60 outdoor minutes daily.

Try forest bathing: Immersing yourself in the woods has scientifically proven benefits for reducing cortisol, anxiety, fatigue and pain sensitivity.

Grow plants: Interacting with live plants cultivates connections with the natural world right at home, reducing stress and anxiety.

Hug loved ones: Hugging releases oxytocin and lowers blood pressure. Aim for at least 8 hugs per day.

Practice kindness: Acts of generosity and kindness elevate oxytocin, serotonin and dopamine improving mood, focus and connection.

Unplug often: Take breaks from social media and screens which can isolate us and increase stress hormones.

Take nature walks: Shinrin-yoku or "forest bathing" reduces cortisol and blood pressure while boosting immunity and energy levels.

Our hormones function best when we prioritize in-person social ties and abundant time in natural settings. Make these a regular part of your routine for optimal hormonal balance.

The lifestyle tips provided in this chapter create an ideal foundation for balanced hormones. Reducing stress, getting quality sleep, exercising, avoiding chemicals and spending time in nature work synergistically to gently nudge your hormones back into alignment.

Chapter 3: Herbal Allies for Hormone Balance

Herbs are nature's medicine, and many have been traditionally used for centuries by herbalists to gently modulate and support healthy hormonal balance. Herbs contain plant compounds that interact with hormone receptors and influence endocrine function. They often provide safer, more holistic hormonal support than synthetic pharmaceuticals.

This chapter provides an overview of key herbs that can be safely used to promote women's hormonal wellness throughout the lifespan. You'll learn how each one specifically helps regulate estrogen, progesterone, testosterone, thyroid hormones, cortisol and other endocrine messengers.

How Herbs Support Hormonal Health

Herbs influence hormones through several mechanisms:

Phytoestrogens: Some herbs contain plant compounds that mimic estrogen in the body. These phytoestrogens bind to estrogen receptors providing gentle hormonal activity without side effects of stronger estrogens. They may also block excess estrogen. Examples are red clover and soy.

Progesterone promoters: Herbs like chasteberry stimulate the pituitary to produce more progesterone naturally. This helps normalize menstrual cycling and reduce PMS.

Hormone precursors: Herbs like tribulus provide building blocks for hormones. Tribulus provides diosgenin which the body can convert to DHEA for supporting testosterone and estrogen.

Hormone receptor regulation: Herbs like hops and ginseng contain ligands that regulate hormone receptor sites, promoting balanced signaling.

Endocrine gland nourishment: Many herbs nourish and tone the endocrine glands like the adrenals and thyroid. Ashwagandha, for example, improves cortisol signaling reducing fatigue.

Hormone metabolism support: Herbs like milk thistle optimize liver function for balanced hormone break down and elimination from the body.

Herbs are also superior to synthetic hormones in that they **contain a spectrum of plant compounds and nutrients** that work synergistically for optimal endocrine health.

Now let's explore some of the top hormone balancing herbs for women.

Key Hormone Balancing Herbs

Chasteberry (Vitex)

Chasteberry, also called vitex, is the most popular herb for supporting women's cycles and hormone balance. It works directly on the pituitary gland to promote healthy progesterone levels. PMS symptoms like breast tenderness, bloating, irregular cycles, acne and irritability improve. It also minimizes hot flashes during perimenopause.

Suggested use: Take 250-500 mg of chasteberry extract each day. Effects build over time. Best taken long term for hormonal regulation.

Maca

Maca root balances estrogen, progesterone and testosterone. It also enhances thyroid health and adrenal function. Maca is beneficial for energy, stamina, reproductive health and emotional wellbeing. It reduces symptoms of menopause like hot flashes and night sweats.

Suggested use: Take 1,500-3,000 mg maca powder daily. Add to smoothies, oatmeal or baked goods. Reduce dose if jittery.

Black Cohosh

Black cohosh has been used for centuries by indigenous peoples of North America. It relieves hot flashes, night sweats, vaginal dryness, mood swings and irritability associated with perimenopause and menopause.

Suggested use: Take 40-80 mg standardized black cohosh extract twice daily. Effects noticed within 6-8 weeks.

Red Clover

Red clover contains phytoestrogens that help block excess estrogen and also replace declining estrogen levels during perimenopause and menopause. This herb improves bone and heart health while reducing menopausal symptoms.

Suggested use: Take 250-500 mg red clover extract daily, or enjoy as tea by steeping blossoms.

Ashwagandha

Ashwagandha is an adaptogenic herb that helps the body adapt to stress. It enhances thyroid function and regulates excess cortisol production resulting in increased energy, improved sleep and clearer thinking.

Suggested use: Take 500 mg high-quality ashwagandha root extract once or twice daily. May cause drowsiness.

Evening Primrose Oil

Evening primrose oil contains high gamma-linolenic acid (GLA) which helps minimize PMS and menopausal symptoms. It also promotes cervical ripening in preparation for labor.

Suggested use: Take 500-1000 mg evening primrose oil supplement daily. Alternatively, consume the oil by adding to salads.

Tribulus

Tribulus provides building blocks for hormones like estrogen, testosterone and DHEA. It enhances libido in women by improving androgen and estrogen balance. Relieves mood swings and anxiety.

Suggested use: Take 750-1500 mg tribulus daily divided into doses. Start with lower dose and increase slowly over 4-6 weeks.

Licorice Root

Licorice boosts low progesterone levels and reduces high testosterone. It also nourishes adrenal glands and balances cortisol. Useful for PCOS, PMS and menopause.

Suggested use: Take 200-400 mg licorice root daily. Do not use with high blood pressure. Limit use to 6 weeks.

Motherwort

Motherwort brings gentle relief from hot flashes, night sweats, heart palpitations, anxiety and insomnia during perimenopause and menopause.

Suggested use: Drink 2-3 cups motherwort tea daily. May also take capsules with 500 mg powdered herb.

This covers some of the top herbal allies for optimizing women's hormonal health. Always **consult an herbalist or healthcare provider before starting herbal regimens**, especially if you have a medical condition or take medications. When used correctly, herbs offer a safer, more holistic alternative to synthetic hormones.

How to Use Herbs Safely and Effectively

Here are some tips for benefiting from hormone balancing herbs:

- **Purchase high-quality herbs** from reputable suppliers. Organic and ethically wildcrafted is best.

- **Talk to an herbalist** for individualized recommendations based on your health history and symptoms.

- **Start slowly** with lower doses and watch for reactions before increasing.

- **Consult a doctor** if combining herbs with medications to ensure safety.

- **Take herbs consistently** for best hormonal balancing results over weeks and months.

- **Make teas** by adding 1 tsp dried herb to 1 cup boiling water, steeping 15 min. Drink 2-3 cups daily.

- **Try tinctures** (alcohol extracts) which absorb quickly. Use 20-40 drops in water 2-3x daily.

- **Add powdered herbs** to smoothies, sprinkled on food or in capsules.

- **Use organic carrier oils** like olive oil to make infused herbal oils for topical use.

Hormone balancing herbs create health from root cause by gently nudging, nourishing and supporting the endocrine system. Make these botanical allies a part of your journey back to hormonal harmony.

Chapter 4: Healing Foods for Hormones

Diet and nutrition exert a powerful influence on hormonal health. Certain foods contain nutrients that promote hormone balance, while other foods can worsen hormone dysfunction. This chapter will explore optimal foods and dietary patterns for supporting healthy hormone levels.

Nutrients for Hormonal Health

A nutritious, whole foods diet provides the vitamins, minerals, antioxidants and plant compounds needed for smooth hormonal regulation. Be sure to get adequate amounts of:

Essential fatty acids like omega-3s found in fatty fish, walnuts, chia and hemp seeds reduce inflammation that contributes to hormone imbalance. Omega-3s also support thyroid hormone function.

Vitamin D from sun exposure, eggs, salmon and mushrooms is needed for modulating estrogen, progesterone, testosterone and thyroid hormones. Deficiency is linked to hormonal cancers and infertility.

Magnesium from leafy greens, nuts, beans and avocados is required for hormone receptor sensitivity and enzymatic reactions that balance hormones. Magnesium calms cortisol.

Zinc found in oysters, nuts, spinach and pumpkin seeds promotes optimal testosterone levels and reproductive health. Zinc is also essential for thyroid hormone balance.

B-vitamins like folate from leafy greens support healthy estrogen metabolism and detoxification. Vitamins B6 and B12 aid hormone balance.

Vitamin C from citrus fruits, kiwi and red bell peppers helps control cortisol levels. Vitamin C also assists liver detoxification of used hormones from the body.

Antioxidants like resveratrol in grapes and lycopene in tomatoes protect hormones and glands from damage by detrimental free radicals exacerbated by stress.

Emphasize these nutrients in your cooking to create meals that support balanced hormones.

An Anti-Inflammatory Diet

Chronic low-grade inflammation disrupts delicate hormonal communication and balance. Following an anti-inflammatory diet minimizes inflammatory triggers:

Eliminate refined carbs and sugars: These spike blood sugar and insulin leading to inflammation and hormone imbalance.

Increase omega-3 rich foods: Omega-3 fatty acids reduce inflammatory compounds like cytokines that interfere with hormones.

Choose organic produce: Pesticides and chemicals in non-organic foods are endocrine disruptors that provoke inflammation.

Reduce red and processed meats: These meats contain arachidonic acid that gets converted into inflammatory prostaglandins.

Avoid hydrogenated oils: Trans fats found in many processed foods trigger inflammatory pathways linked to hormone dysfunction.

Reduce caffeine and alcohol: These stimulants release stress hormones and increase inflammatory markers.

Stay hydrated: Drink at least 64 ounces of filtered water daily to flush out inflammation-causing toxins.

Choosing anti-inflammatory foods like colorful produce, herbs and spices, lean proteins, nuts and olive oil provides the basis for balanced hormones and optimal health.

Manage Blood Sugar

When blood sugar spikes, so does insulin, the hormone that lowers high blood glucose. Excess insulin disrupts the ovaries, endocrine glands and hormone receptor sites. Stabilizing blood sugar is key:

Eat smaller, frequent meals with a combination of protein, healthy fats and complex carbs to balance blood sugar all day.

Avoid refined grains and added sugars that cause insulin to spike then crash blood sugar levels.

Choose whole food carbs like sweet potatoes, quinoa, beans, oats and non-starchy veggies to minimize blood sugar fluctuations.

Increase dietary fiber from vegetables, nuts, seeds and whole grains which helps regulate blood sugar rises after meals.

Exercise regularly to increase insulin receptor sensitivity and keep blood glucose balanced at healthy levels.

Drink cinnamon tea daily since cinnamon helps reduce and stabilize blood sugar especially after high carb meals.

Following a low glycemic diet that minimizes blood sugar spikes and dips prevents hormonal mayhem.

Phytoestrogenic Foods

Phytoestrogens are plant compounds that mimic estrogen in the body. Foods rich in phytoestrogens can help ease hormone imbalance symptoms like hot flashes, mood swings, vaginal dryness and irregular cycles by lightly binding to estrogen receptors. Phytoestrogenic foods include:

Soy foods like tofu, tempeh, miso and edamame contain isoflavone phytoestrogens that balance hormones.

Flaxseeds offer lignan phytoestrogens that mimic estrogen while blocking excess estrogen activity.

Sesame seeds provide phytoestrogens and promote progesterone production for cycle balance.

Alfalfa sprouts are a rich source of plant estrogens helpful for menopause and fertility.

Dried fruits like dates, prunes, cherries and apricots are high in phytoestrogens.

Herbs like oregano, thyme, basil, parsley, sage and mint contain phytoestrogenic compounds.

Enjoy these healing phytoestrogenic foods daily as part of a balanced diet. But those with estrogen-receptor positive cancers need to avoid phytoestrogenic foods.

Sample Hormone Balancing Meal Plan

Here is an ideal day of anti-inflammatory, blood sugar friendly, hormone nourishing meals:

Breakfast: Scrambled eggs with wilted spinach, avocado and rye toast. Pineapple chunks.

Snack: Homemade trail mix with walnuts, pumpkin seeds, goji berries. Green tea.

Lunch: Grilled salmon over quinoa pilaf with roasted Brussels sprouts and carrots.

Snack: Celery sticks with almond butter. Kiwifruit.

Dinner: Baked chicken with sweet potato and roasted broccoli. Salad with chickpeas, beets, sunflower seeds and balsamic dressing.

Dessert: Dark chocolate covered strawberries. Chamomile tea.

This provides balanced macronutrients, anti-inflammatory foods, blood sugar friendly carbs and an array of hormones supporting nutrients. Use it as a template and get creative adapting recipes to your tastes!

The optimal diet for hormone health focuses on anti-inflammatory whole foods that stabilize blood sugar. Incorporating phytoestrogenic foods and key micronutrients provides additional endocrine nourishing benefits.

Chapter 5: Supplements for Hormonal Balance

While diet should always be the foundation, certain supplements can provide concentrated nourishment to support balanced hormones when needs are not fully met through foods alone. Let's explore key micronutrients, adaptogens and other beneficial supplements for hormone health.

Vitamins, Minerals and Omegas

Magnesium relaxes muscles for less painful periods, lowers cortisol and helps balance blood sugar. Take 400 mg daily.

Vitamin D3 enhances hormone receptor function and modulates estrogen metabolism. Take 2000-5000 IU daily or get 15 min midday sun.

B-complex provides crucial B vitamins like choline and folate for proper estrogen detoxification. Take a quality B-complex supplement.

Omega-3 fish oils like cod liver oil or krill oil combat inflammation that disturbs hormone pathways. Take 3000 mg EPA/DHA daily.

Iodine ensures adequate thyroid hormone synthesis and metabolism. Kelp tablets provide 150-300 mcg iodine.

Zinc promotes hormone receptor binding, menstrual health and modulates testosterone. Take 15-30 mg zinc picolinate daily.

Selenium enhances thyroid hormone conversion and protects the thyroid. Brazil nuts offer selenium. Take 200 mcg supplement.

Vitamin E improves hormonal balance and reduces hot flashes, night sweats and vaginal dryness during menopause. Take 400 IU mixed tocopherols.

Iron prevents anemia-related fatigue and thyroid problems in women. Take gentle iron bisglycinate tablets or eat iron-rich foods.

Cover your nutritional bases with a high quality multivitamin/mineral that includes these key nutrients. Add individual supplements like magnesium, omega-3s and vitamin D3 based on your specific needs.

Adaptogenic Herbs

Adaptogens enhance the body's resiliency to stress and promote hormone balance. Consider these hormonal superheros:

Ashwagandha regulates thyroid hormone, reduces excess cortisol, improves insulin sensitivity and balances testosterone and estrogen. Take 500 mg daily.

Maca root nourishes the hypothalamus-pituitary axis to balance sex hormones and cortisol. Take 1-2 grams daily.

Rhodiola optimizes cortisol rhythms and protects thyroid hormones during stress. Take 100-200 mg standardized extract daily.

Holy basil counteracts elevated cortisol, regulates insulin and lowers anxiety. Take 500 mg daily as tea or supplement.

Panax ginseng alleviates menopausal symptoms, modulates cortisol response, boosts estrogen and stabilizes blood sugar. Take 100-500 mg standardized extract up to twice daily.

Licorice root nourishes adrenals, balances cortisol and boosts progesterone. Limit use to 6 weeks due to side effects. Take 400 mg daily.

Using adaptogens alongside targeted herbs results in a powerfully supportive protocol for achieving hormonal homeostasis.

Other Hormone Balancing Supplements

DHEA replaces declining DHEA hormone common during perimenopause and beyond. May help improve mood, sleep, libido and energy. Take 25-50 mg DHEA.

DIM helps metabolize excess estrogen and manage estrogen dominance. May also boost testosterone. Take 100-200 mg DIM supplement daily.

Calcium d-glucarate aids liver detoxification and estrogen metabolism. Take 200-500 mg daily.

Saw palmetto blocks excessive testosterone at receptor sites and optimizes hormonal balance. Take 160 mg daily.

CoQ10 enhances egg quality and ovarian function. Take 100-200 mg per day along with fertility treatments.

Probiotics reduce gut bacterial imbalance contributing to hormonal issues in some women. Consume probiotic foods and/or take 50 billion CFU probiotic supplement daily.

Discuss specific supplement recommendations with your healthcare provider to identify optimal choices based on your lab results and symptoms. Use supplements judiciously for a few months until diet and lifestyle habits improve.

The supplements highlighted in this chapter offer concentrated hormonal assistance. However, they should complement, not replace, a healthy diet, active lifestyle, stress management and hormone balancing herbs for full restorative results.

Chapter 6: Natural Solutions for Specific Hormonal Stages and Issues

Now that we've covered lifestyle tips, healing foods, herbs and supplements for overall hormone balance, let's explore targeted natural solutions for specific hormonal stages and common women's health conditions.

Herbal Remedies for PMS, Menstrual Issues

For most women, hormonal shifts each month can result in PMS symptoms like breast tenderness, bloating, headaches, anxiety, food cravings and irritability. Heavy, painful periods with cramping and irregular cycles can also occur. Here are some natural remedies:

Chasteberry regulates menstrual cycles and promotes progesterone production to minimize PMS and irregular periods. Take 400 mg daily.

Dong quai reduces cramping by improving uterine circulation. Make dong quai tea or take capsules. Do not use if you have fibroids.

Ginger decreases prostaglandin production to ease menstrual cramps. Drink ginger tea or take capsules with meals.

Magnesium glycinate relaxes muscle tension and calms the nervous system to alleviate anxiety, breast tenderness, headaches and trouble sleeping related to PMS. Take 300 mg daily.

Vitex combined with **black cohosh** improves PMS symptoms like breast pain, acne, headaches and mood swings in clinical studies.

Maca root helps balance estrogen and progesterone which regulates cycles and reduces PMS. Take 1-2 grams daily.

Evening primrose oil provides essential fatty acids to minimize breast tenderness and hormonal headaches. Take 1-2 grams daily.

Avoid caffeine, alcohol, sugar and refined carbs which can worsen PMS. Getting enough sleep, exercise and stress reduction also helps.

Natural Menopause Relief

Shifting hormone levels during perimenopause and menopause cause symptoms like hot flashes, night sweats, vaginal dryness, trouble sleeping, irritability, brain fog and disinterest in sex. Here are some soothing natural remedies:

Black cohosh greatly reduces hot flashes, night sweats and irritability. Studies confirm its efficacy. Take 40-80 mg twice daily.

Maca root balances hormones while boosting energy and sex drive. Take 1500-3000 mg daily.

Flaxseeds contain phytoestrogens that minimize hot flashes. Sprinkle 2 Tbs ground flax daily on foods or in water.

Vitamin E 400 IU daily decreases hot flashes and vaginal dryness. Choose natural mixed tocopherols.

Evening primrose oil provides essential fatty acids to moderate menopausal symptoms. Take 500-1000 mg daily.

Acupuncture successfully reduces hot flashes and night sweats for many women. Get 8-12 treatments.

Meditation is proven to reduce menopausal symptoms by lowering cortisol, blood pressure and stress. Sit quietly for 10-20 minutes daily.

Be patient as you allow herbs, diet and lifestyle changes to promote hormonal equilibrium and a easier passage through "the change".

Natural Fibroid Remedies

Uterine fibroids are non-cancerous growths in the uterus affecting up to 80% of women by age 50. Fibroids cause symptoms like heavy menstrual bleeding, pelvic pain and pressure. Here are some natural ways to shrink fibroids:

Vitex helps prevent new fibroid growth by normalizing estrogen and progesterone balance. Take 400 mg daily.

Ginger decreases inflammation and prostaglandin production which reduces fibroid pain and heavy bleeding. Drink ginger tea daily and cook with fresh ginger.

Turmeric provides the powerful anti-inflammatory compound curcumin shown to shrink uterine fibroids. Take a curcumin supplement or use turmeric liberally in cooking.

Green tea contains epigallocatechin gallate (EGCG) which prevents the growth of fibroid cells. Drink 2-3 cups of green tea daily.

Fasting gives the body a break from excess estrogen which encourages fibroid growth. Do a fresh juice fast or intermittent fasting for 1-2 days a month.

Calcium d-glucarate supports the liver's elimination of excess estrogen contributing to fibroids. Take 200-500 mg daily.

Acupuncture increases circulation, reduces fibroid size and alleviates painful periods. Get regular fertility-focused treatments.

Natural PCOS Management

PCOS leads to excess testosterone, absent periods, infertility, acne and hair growth on the face and body. Making the following lifestyle changes can help restore hormonal balance:

Follow a PCOS diet - Emphasize complex carbs, lean protein, healthy fats and fiber. Avoid sugar, refined grains and dairy which worsen symptoms.

Take inositol - This B vitamin improves insulin sensitivity and fertility. Take 1200-4000 mg daily.

Exercise regularly - Try interval training as this reduces testosterone and insulin resistance that contribute to PCOS.

Manage stress - High cortisol exacerbates PCOS. Try light walking, meditation and adaptogens like ashwagandha to lower excess cortisol.

See an acupuncturist - Acupuncture helps regulate menstrual cycles, minimize hair growth, aids fertility and improves PCOS symptoms.

Take saw palmetto - This herbal anti-androgen inhibits the conversion of testosterone at receptor sites. Take 160 mg daily.

Use spearmint tea bags - Spearmint tea reduces hirsutism and androgen levels in women with PCOS. Drink spearmint tea twice daily.

Try guava leaf tea - The antispasmodic actions help induce menstrual cycles. Drink guava tea daily.

With a multifaceted, natural approach hormonal balance and regular cycles can be restored in women with PCOS.

The holistic protocols in this chapter provide gentler alternatives to medications for woman-specific hormone issues throughout the lifecycle. As you now know, you have many natural options to find hormone harmony once again!

Conclusion

Our delicate hormonal balance profoundly impacts mental and physical wellbeing. Yet many women struggle with the effects of hormonal chaos – irregular cycles, infertility, fatigue, low libido, weight gain, insomnia, anxiety and more.

The good news is that you now have a wealth of natural tools to restore harmony to your hormones. As we've explored, lifestyle changes, healing foods, herbs and supplements can gently nudge your hormones back into alignment without the need for synthetic hormones or medications.

This book provided solutions to target hormonal health from multiple angles. You learned about the roles hormones play in keeping the body functioning optimally. We covered how to identify symptoms of hormonal imbalance, and explored root causes like chronic stress, blood sugar dysregulation, gut issues and toxins.

Lifestyle fixes like managing stress through meditation and adaptogens offer foundational hormone support. Adequate sleep, regular exercise and spending time in nature also emerged as non-negotiables. An anti-inflammatory, whole foods diet stabilizes blood sugar and supplies hormone-nourishing nutrients.

Herbal allies like chasteberry, maca and black cohosh provide safe, botanical assistance in modulating estrogen, testosterone, cortisol and more. Carefully selected supplements fill any nutritional gaps interfering with hormone health.

Then we applied natural solutions to specific issues plaguing women – PMS, infertility, menstrual problems, menopause, fibroids, PCOS and beyond. You now have evidence-based natural tools to move through each hormonal stage gracefully.

I hope this book has outlined a clear path to find balance once again. Be patient with yourself on the journey. Your body wants to find homeostasis. Support it by consistently implementing the diet, lifestyle and holistic practices shared within these pages.

You have the power to nourish your hormones back to harmony the natural way – without synthetic hormones or medications. Here's to reclaiming optimal energy, stable moods, restful sleep, resilient health and feminine radiance!

About the Author

Dr. Omolola Habib is a certified health and wellness coach specializing in women's hormonal health, functional medicine and herbal remedies; she also holds a license as a Naturopathic Doctor.

Dr. Habib's personal struggles with PCOS, endometriosis and thyroid issues earlier in life ignited her passion for assisting women in discovering natural solutions to restore hormonal balance. Failing to find relief through conventional medicine herself, she explored the realms of naturopathy, nutrition and herbs; these pursuits ultimately revolutionized her health.

Dr. Habib, utilizing an integrative approach that combines natural modalities such as nutrition, botanicals, acupuncture and bioidentical hormones when necessary with the finest conventional medicine; now imparts her wealth of personal experience and clinical knowledge to patients in her private practice.

Dr. Habib passionately empowers women to seize control of their hormonal health, encouraging them to harness the power of natural remedies for achieving balance and enhancing overall wellbeing. She finds great pleasure in formulating custom herbal remedies and divulging her recipes for meals that promote optimal health.

Outside of her patient interactions, she engages in activities such as hiking, gardening or indulging in Portland's food scene. Dr. Habib aspires for this book to not only provide enlightenment but also serve as an inspirational guide on your personal quest towards hormonal balance.